Calm in the Storm

A Compassionate Survival Guide
for PANS/PANDAS Parents in the Worst of It
(from a Mom Who Has Been in the Trenches)

Written and Illustrated by Andrea Phillips

First Edition.

TABLE OF CONTENTS

Introduction

If you're reading this, I want to say something before anything else:

You are still here, and that means something. Also, you are not alone.

I wrote this short book with the hope that it may help someone else who is going through what I've gone through.

This work, loving a child through PANS/PANDAS, is not parenting in the way most people understand it. It is walking with someone you love through fire. It is learning to live inside a storm. It is holding a flashlight for someone who can't always see you, or even themselves. It is advocating endlessly. It is having to explain over and over why your child is different, why you can't participate in things the way most people can. It is defending your nontraditional parenting because this illness requires flexibility. It is incredibly isolating. I want you to know that I see you. All of us who have experienced this see you.
Some days it gets so dark, you lose your sense of time. Your sense of self. You wonder if there is any way through. I have been there.
There were moments I did not know if we would survive. It also felt like the help that should have come... didn't.

But here we are. Still here.

This little book was born in that space: the in-between, where there are no easy answers, but still somehow there's presence. There's a sliver of light that gets in, even when it feels like everything has gone dark.

You won't find any cures here. Just words for when you are struggling. Simple scripts, grounding tools, offerings of comfort, ways to stay with your child and yourself when everything inside you is unraveling.

I wrote this because it's the little book I wish I'd had ten years ago when my child was just beginning to show symptoms, which no one in our family understood. I hope it helps someone else feel a little less alone.

There is a path through. It doesn't always look like healing in the way you hoped. Sometimes, it looks like a brief moment of respite or joy. A glimmer of recognition in their eyes after months of blank stares. An emergency that you survived. A moment where you remember you're still human, too, and you laugh a little at something. Acknowledgement from someone who truly understands.

You don't have to be calm all the time. You don't actually have to fix it. You just have to keep showing up with love for your child and compassion for yourself. This little book is here to help you do that.

You are not alone in this important, brutal work.

With deep respect,
Andrea Kresge Phillips | Juniper Moon Colors

Before We Begin

The following sections highlight common themes in PANS/PANDAS, patterns I've seen again and again, and ones I've lived through myself. There's no one-size-fits-all solution for this journey, but I believe there are nuggets of wisdom here that may resonate, guide, or simply help you feel less alone.

At the time of writing, my child is 20. I consider myself a seasoned veteran, not a title I ever imagined. And we're still not finished. The healing process is ongoing. But with some distance and hindsight, I can say this:

I've come to know myself in astonishing ways.
I've grown in strength, awareness, patience, and compassion, and my whole family was pushed to expand in directions we never would've chosen, but that changed us deeply. There is growth in struggle. Something new is forged under duress.

Try to think of it like that, because it's true.

Take what serves you from these pages, and leave what doesn't. And if you know another parent navigating this storm, feel free to share it with them. Sometimes, even a few supportive words can change the shape of a day.

Each topic includes a section called *Anchoring Phrases:* simple, supportive things you can say when you're feeling overwhelmed or unsure how to respond.

Please feel free to use them, adapt them, or create your own. What matters most is that your words come from a calm, steady place and are tailored to your child's age, needs, and developmental level. Think of these as starting points, not scripts.

What Is PANS/PANDAS?

PANS (Pediatric Acute-onset Neuropsychiatric Syndrome) and PANDAS (Pediatric Autoimmune Neuropsychiatric Disorders Associated with Streptococcal infections) are forms of **autoimmune encephalitis**. That means the immune system, after an infection or other trigger, mistakenly attacks parts of the brain, especially regions that regulate mood, movement, behavior, and decision-making.

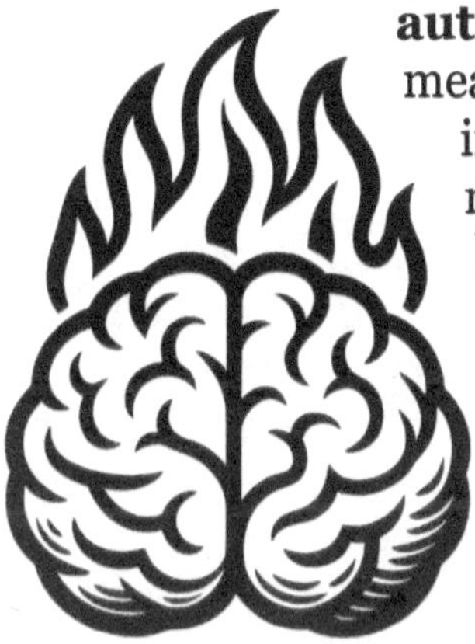

This brain inflammation can lead to sudden or gradual onset of severe symptoms like OCD, anxiety, rage, tics, eating restrictions, sleep disturbance, cognitive decline, or even hallucinations and psychosis.

Although the name suggests an "acute" onset, many children experience a slow-burning progression that is easily misdiagnosed or overlooked for years.

This is **not psychological** in origin. It is **biological and inflammatory,** a nervous system in crisis. And when treated at the root, healing is possible.

If you're like me, no matter how many times you've explained this to someone you may still forget the details. You can refer back to this section in the future if you need a concise definition for anyone - family, friends, doctors, etc.

When OCD Is the First Sign

Anxiety, rituals, and rage: what we thought was behavior was actually brain inflammation.

I'm starting with this topic, because OCD is usually one of the first things parents notice, and also one of the most life-altering aspects of PANS/PANDAS. It affects the entire family. OCD in PANS/PANDAS doesn't always look like the stereotypical hand-washing or checking behaviors. Sometimes it's loud, scary, or deeply irrational. Sometimes it shows up as intrusive thoughts, compulsive confessing, rituals that make no sense to anyone else, or a desperate need for reassurance over and over again.

It can feel impossible to reason with, because it *is* impossible to reason with. OCD is not logical. These are brain-based symptoms. And when they flare, they take over.

OCD doesn't always look like fear of germs. It can also show up as **fixations, compulsive eating, hoarding, counting, or collecting.** It can manifest as **scrupulosity,** a painful fixation on morality or spiritual concepts. The rituals might not make sense to anyone but the child.

The line between behavior and symptoms can get blurry. But one of the most important anchors you can hold onto is this:

It's OCD, not your child.

Sometimes it helps to give the OCD a name so everyone can separate it from the real person underneath.
You could call it *The Bully.*

When things got hard, we'd say: *"That's just The Bully again."*

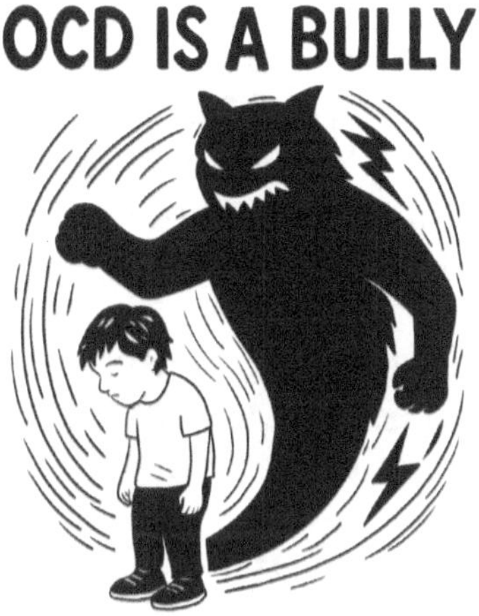

Because that's exactly what it is, a bully.
Your child is being bullied by their own mind.

As a parent, this can be one of the hardest things to witness.
Your child might say things they don't mean, do things that scare you, or get trapped in thought loops that bring both of you to tears.

Sometimes OCD demands compliance from everyone in the household. It can manipulate, threaten, or punish. It can become a kind of tyrant in your home.

You are not a bad parent if you feel exhausted or angry or scared by it.

Sometimes OCD wins.
You give in just to keep the peace, to avoid a meltdown, to make it through the moment. Don't blame yourself. And don't let anyone else make you feel ashamed.

I've talked to so many parents over the years who've had to make constant exceptions and concessions just to survive the day. OCD demands that. It wears you down. It corners you. It asks too much.

It's disheartening, it's exhausting, and saying *it's difficult* doesn't even come close.

You're not alone. So many of us have been there. Sometimes surviving *is* the win.

The truth is, no one is really prepared for what OCD can look like in a child with PANS/PANDAS. But you *can* get through it. You can hold your child with compassion *and* set boundaries with the OCD. You can learn to speak to your child, not the symptom.

You are allowed to grieve the changes this brings to your family. And you are allowed to protect your own mental health in the process.

Our Experience with OCD

OCD was one of the very first symptoms to appear for us and one of the most misunderstood.

In hindsight, it was an early sign that my child's brain was inflamed and struggling. But at the time, none of us knew that. My child was 10, and the first thing we saw was Contamination OCD. It started with little things: fears about germs, touching certain objects, rituals around cleanliness. Everyone around us, including teachers, therapists and extended family, treated it like a *behavior problem*. Since we already had an autism diagnosis, every quirk or problem was attributed to that. Because of this, we totally missed PANS as a possibility for five more years.

That's a trap many families fall into. OCD is one of the most visible symptoms of PANS/PANDAS, but the disorder itself often goes unrecognized. The default path is standard OCD treatment: therapy and medications. That's not inherently wrong. CBT and SSRIs help many people, but when the root issue is autoimmune brain inflammation, those tools alone might not even scratch the surface.

We tried several SSRIs. None of them helped. Some made things worse. The side effects were awful. Through that process, we even discovered that the coloring and fillers in the pills were triggering reactions. The worst one for us was Luvox, supposedly the gold standard for OCD, yet it sent my child into a near-psychotic tailspin.

This just goes to show: **every kid is different**.

We had a psychiatrist who spent maybe five minutes with our child. Most of the actual prescribing was done by nurse practitioners. Meanwhile, the deeper cause, PANS, was going unaddressed, and my child was spiraling.

Eventually, we came to understand that **OCD wasn't the main problem**. It was a **symptom:** evidence that my child's brain was inflamed, misfiring, and stuck. We call it having a *sticky mind*. And until we addressed the underlying medical issues, the OCD never really budged.

A Word About Meanness

OCD is an anxiety disorder, and anxiety often shows up in unexpected ways. Sometimes it looks like panic or avoidance. But sometimes it looks like **rage, cruelty, or meanness.**

It took us a long time to understand this.

There were years when our child was triggered by things that made no sense to anyone else: my breath, the appearance of my feet, the texture of my voice, the sound of chewing. Their reactions felt harsh, even vicious. And because I was the primary caregiver, I bore the brunt of it. I felt crushed and abused.

But what I eventually came to understand is this:
It wasn't personal. It was neurological.

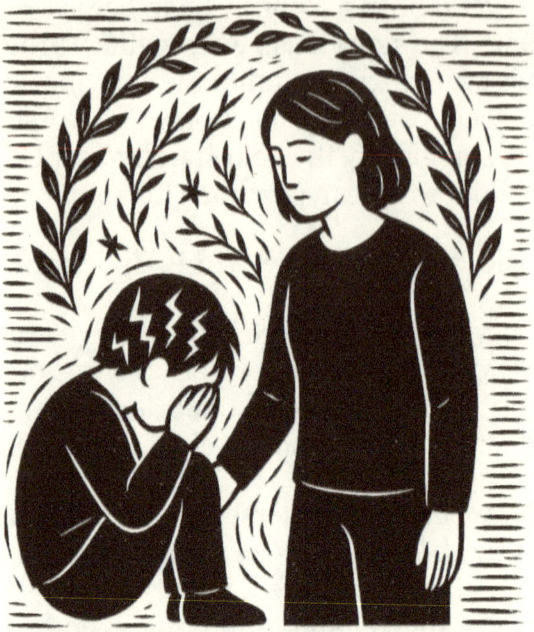

IT'S NOT PERSONAL, IT'S NEUROLOGICAL.

Their brain was inflamed. Their anxiety was through the roof. And their reactions, while painful to witness and endure, were not reflections of their true self or their love for me. It was just their brain on fire, desperately trying to find control in a world that felt unsafe.

This doesn't mean we don't set boundaries or protect ourselves, it means we understand the nuance.

This is a child in distress,

not a child being bad.

This is what anxiety-driven OCD can look like.

If your child's behavior feels cruel or targeted, you are not weak for feeling hurt. And you are not alone. Many PANS/PANDAS parents experience this. You are loving your child through something *very few people understand.*

If They Could Do Better, They Would

This has been one of our family's most-used mantras. That simple truth anchored us through years of confusion and heartbreak. Because honestly, what kid *wants* to be stuck in a 20-minute handwashing loop until their skin is raw? What kid *wants* to take a three-hour shower and still feel dirty? What kid wants to have a public meltdown that traumatizes everyone? Ours didn't.

Our child wore gloves to touch nearly everything for about five straight years, not because they were seeking attention, not because they were being dramatic, but because their brain told them it wasn't safe not to. This is just one example. I am not even going to share some of the more personal or shocking things.

This is what PANS/PANDAS OCD can look like. It's not rebellion, it's not manipulation, it's a child trapped in a body that feels out of control, desperately trying to find a way to feel okay.

Remembering that they *would do better if they could* can help us meet them with the compassion and steadiness they need, especially when everything in us is overwhelmed and exhausted.

For the Doubters in Your Life

OCD is not a parenting problem. It is not a discipline problem.

You cannot punish it away, reason it away, or "consequence" it into submission. Trying to discipline OCD out of a child can actually make things worse, because it increases shame, fear, and the compulsive drive to hide symptoms. What kids need is understanding, not punishment. Boundaries, yes, but also compassion, safety, and the right support for what's really going on in the brain.

If you're dealing with family members, friends, or professionals who insist this is a discipline issue, or who accuse you of being enmeshed or codependent, feel free to share this:

What you're seeing is not the result of poor parenting, lack of discipline, or enmeshment. This is a medical condition affecting the brain. PANS/ PANDAS can cause OCD, rages, regressions, and other neurological symptoms that are often misinterpreted as behavioral or emotional issues. Standard parenting techniques don't work here, not because the parent is weak or codependent, but because the child is *ill*. The most effective approach is medical treatment, nervous system support, and trauma-informed care. If you want to help, start by believing the parents, not blaming them.

What this child needs is compassion—not tough love.

You can't push or punish a child out of brain inflammation. Healing comes through safety, trust, and the right medical care not shame or force.

If you don't have an official PANDAS diagnosis, tell your family members it is neurodivergence. The same things apply. You can't discipline a brain type into compliance.

The First to Arrive, the Last to Leave

In many cases, **OCD is the first symptom to appear and the last one to go.** It can linger long after other symptoms begin to improve. That's not meant to scare you; it's meant to prepare you.

As the saying goes:

"To be forewarned is to be forearmed."

Knowing this ahead of time can help you pace yourself, build resilience, and understand that slow progress is still progress.

OCD can feel like a battle. A relentless, shape-shifting opponent. It helps to **connect with parenting groups,** both those specific to PANS and those for OCD in general. There's a wealth of knowledge, support, and shared experience out there.

But it's also important to remember:
Not every child with OCD has PANS.
Many kids with primary OCD respond very well to standard treatments: SSRIs, CBT, ERP (exposure response prevention), and intensive programs like those at Rogers or similar clinics.

A child with PANS may not.

Why? Because a brain in the midst of inflammation can't always tolerate that kind of therapy. **Before exposure work or behavioral interventions can be effective, the brain needs to calm.** Medical treatment and nervous system support must come first.

So don't feel discouraged if your child isn't able to do what others in OCD support groups are doing. You're not failing, you're just dealing with a **different root cause** and healing is still possible.

Anchoring Phrases for OCD Moments

When OCD takes hold, it can feel like your child has been pulled into a storm. These are phrases you can reach for, words that don't fix everything, but help steady the moment.

- "I see you're really stuck right now. I'm here. I still love you."
- "This isn't you, it's the OCD talking. Let's take a breath together."
- "You don't have to explain it all. I know it feels urgent, but you are safe."
- "You are not bad. Your brain is just sending the wrong signals right now."
- "I know it's hard to stop. I'll help you through it, one step at a time."
- "Let's get through this wave. You've done it before. You can do it again."
- "I'm not mad at you. I know you don't want to feel this way either."
- "You're not alone. We're on the same team."
- "You don't have to do the compulsion. I'll sit with you while we wait." (Or alternatively, you stay with them while they do the compulsion, then discuss it afterward. Sometimes preventing them from doing it can worsen issues in complex ways. This is so tricky. I am no expert, just a mom that's been through it).

When They Refuse to Go to School

Not Defiant. Not Lazy. Just Trying to Survive.

School refusal is a misunderstood symptom of PANS/PANDAS. It may start suddenly after an illness, a trauma, or a flare, and quickly become a source of conflict, shame, and panic for the whole family. You may feel self-conscious about what the school will think. You may feel like a failure.

They might cry, rage, hide, or go completely limp. They might scream that they're dying. They might seem fine until the last minute, then crumble. You may try rewards, logic, schedules, threats, begging, accommodations. None of it works because this isn't defiance, this is survival, and their nervous system is saying: "I cannot go."

Anchoring Phrases (for Them)

- "I believe you. Something in your body is saying 'no,' and I trust that."
- "School seems to be causing you distress. I believe you."
- "You're not in trouble. You're not bad. You're overwhelmed."
- "Let's figure this out together. I'm not leaving you alone in this."
- "You are more important to me than school."
- "We can find other ways to learn when you're ready."

Anchoring Phrases (For You, the Parent)

- "This is not a parenting failure. This is a neurological crisis."
- "I am allowed to protect my child from systems that don't understand."
- "It is okay to stop forcing what is harming them."

- "We are not behind, we are on a different timeline."
- "I can advocate without explaining everything to everyone."

Optional Steps (When You Have Capacity)

- Track patterns (certain teachers, classrooms, foods, infections?)
- Request a temporary IEP or 504 plan even for homeschool
- Consider medical homebound status or alternative programs
- Keep the pressure low: stability first, education second. There is lots of time to learn.
- Validate feelings: "School feels too much right now, I get that."

When You're Not Sure What's Real

Sometimes it's hard to tell:
Is this a flare or avoidance? Is it infection or anxiety? Is my child manipulating or breaking down?
That confusion doesn't make you a bad parent. It makes you an *attuned one*.
When the lines blur, ask:

- "What happens in their body when school is mentioned?" *(Does their face change? Do they freeze, tremble, lash out, have nausea or intestinal distress?)*
- "Does this reaction feel like a *pattern* or a *performance*?" *(Even dramatic behavior can be regulation-driven, not manipulative.)*
- "What happens *after* we push them to go?" *(Do they escalate? Collapse? Get sick or shut down?)*
- "What are they like when they get home?" *(Are they cheerful, depleted, dysregulated, or unable to function?)*

- “What do I feel in my own body when I see their resistance?” *(Fear? Doubt? Sadness? A subtle knowing? Trust those cues. You have intuition about your child. It’s there.)*

And finally:

“What if I believed them today? What would that change?”

Maybe everything. Or maybe nothing. But believing them today builds trust. It tells your child, *I see you. I’m listening*. Even if it turns out they *could* have managed school today, choosing to believe them doesn’t mean you’re naive; it means you’re present.

You are allowed to get it wrong. Connection matters more than perfection. When you slow down and observe instead of rushing to fix, your ability to understand what’s really going on will deepen. Discernment isn’t immediate. It grows from being present and observing.

We ended up switching to **cyber school**, and it was a tremendous relief. As time went on and the illness worsened, we transitioned to **traditional homeschooling**, and eventually to **unschooling**. I’m not necessarily recommending that path, but for us, it was a necessity. Our child simply couldn’t manage anything else.

You can get creative with schooling. There are some wonderful online options now, and every U.S. state has a system in place for homeschooling families. If you’re considering this, I highly recommend visiting askpauline.com for state-by-state info and support.

If you're outside the U.S., I can’t speak to your legal process, but just know this: **It’s not wrong or bad if your child needs alternative schooling.**

Meeting your child where they are is not failure, it's wisdom.

This section is about permission to slow down, to trust what you're seeing, to resist the story that school refusal means your child is broken or you are weak.

Anchoring Phrases for Disapproving Family Members

- "We're doing what's best for *our* child, even if it looks different from what others expect."
- "This isn't about spoiling or enabling. It's about responding to a medical or neurological condition that affects the brain."
- "I'm not asking for permission. I'm asking for respect."
- "If you can't offer support, I at least need space and acceptance."
- "You don't have to agree with us to show compassion."
- "We're following the advice of specialists who understand PANS/PANDAS, not outdated ideas about discipline or education."
- "We've tried the conventional route. Now we're doing what's actually helping."
- "You may not see the whole picture, but we're in it every day and we're making the best choices we can."

When Your Child Goes Silent

Shutdown, Selective Mutism, or Wordlessness During a Flare

Silence can be terrifying. It can feel like your child has disappeared inside themselves. You may want to reach for them with questions, to pull them back with logic or comfort. But in this state, speech can feel overwhelming, dangerous, or even impossible for them. However, a reassuring word may also make all the difference.

This is a time to regulate your own nervous system first. Speak less, soften more. Trust that connection is still happening through your presence even without words.

There was a period of time when my child was having seizures. They were 16-years-old at the time and it was utterly terrifying. We were up all night together while the rest of the family slept, and so I navigated it alone. There was one night when I was holding my seizing child and after it passed the only words that cut through the fog were lyrics to their favorite song. I started to sing it and then I heard their voice weakly saying the lyrics with me. Get creative if you need to. Try something like that. It lets them know you are there.

Hopefully your situation isn't that extreme and you can talk to your child who may be lost in the world of brain inflammation and unable to articulate what they think and feel.

Here are some ideas for ways to get through.

Anchoring Phrases (No Reply Needed)

- "It's okay if you can't talk. I understand. I'm here for you."

- "You don't have to explain anything. Just breathe. I'm here."
- "Even if you're quiet, I know you're still in there."
- "This part will pass. You don't have to do anything."
- "Your brain and body might be tired. You're allowed to rest."
- "I'll stay close. You don't need to say a word."
- If they have a favorite comfort show, try putting it on and watching it together. See if you can get them to smile, laugh, or interact with it in some small way. For us it's still *SpongeBob*.

One-Way Communication Tools

If your child can't speak but wants to express something, offer low-effort options:

- A notebook or small whiteboard to draw or write.
- Printed cards that say "I'm overwhelmed," "I need space," "I need help."
- A weighted item or comfort object to hand you when they need connection
- A gentle squeeze system: one squeeze = yes, two = no.
- If your child has a phone, text each other. I downloaded Discord for this purpose (and am still trying to get my Gen X brain to understand it).
- Create a code word. When my child was overwhelmed or heading into what we called the "red zone," we decided they could say one word, and I'd know it was time to shift gears, offer space, reduce demands, or change the environment. For a while, that word was *"ointment"* because it made us both laugh.

For When You Feel Desperate for a Response, But Don't Get One

- "Right now, I don't need you to be okay. I just want you to know I'm here."
- "I love you in every state. Even the quiet ones."
- "This silence isn't permanent. We've made it through before."
- "I'll wait until you're ready to talk. I'll be here."
- Gentle touch can help. Putting your hand on their head, a light back massage, a comforting hug. On the other hand, some kids don't want to be touched at all. You know your child best.

Remember: they will come back.
This is an illness *and it's treatable*. The path forward may feel overwhelming or mysterious, and the treatments can be complex, even exhausting. But healing is possible. There are many modalities to explore.

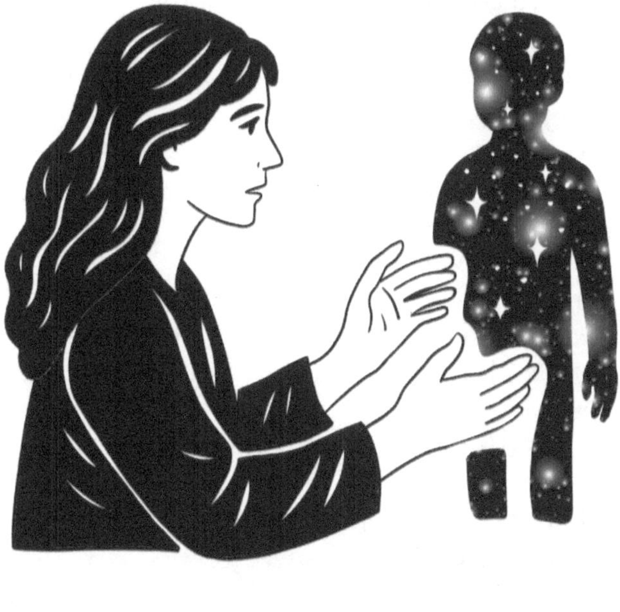

When Food Seems to Make Them Worse

Inflamed Bodies, Impossible Choices, and the Food Struggle

Food becomes one of the most painful battlegrounds in chronic neuroinflammatory illness. What should be nourishing becomes confusing, inflammatory, even terrifying. A simple meal can turn into a meltdown, a migraine, a day in bed, even a psychotic episode.
You may start to dread feeding your child. You may feel like the food is poisoning them, but you're the one giving it. You try gluten-free, dairy-free, low histamine, low oxalate, no dyes, organic only. Nothing feels safe. Everything feels suspect.
And yet... they have to eat.

Anchoring Phrases (for Them)

- "I believe you when you say you feel bad after you eat."
- "We're going to figure this out together. You're not in trouble."
- "Your body is giving us clues. We're going to listen, not panic."
- "We can go slow. You don't have to eat anything that feels unsafe right now."
- "You're not bad for not being hungry. Your body is working really hard."
- "I know you really want to eat that but it's best to wait and have a treat later. Your body needs to heal a bit first."

Anchoring Phrases (for You, the Parent)

- "I am not harming my child by feeding them. I am doing my best."

- "This is not just picky eating. This is the body in survival mode."
- "Even if I can't solve the food puzzle yet, I can offer safety and consistency."
- "It's normal that I feel stressed about this. This is grief. This is exhaustion."
- "I can give healthier options, not out of control, but out of compassion."

Patterns to Watch

- Do symptoms worsen after certain food groups (gluten, dairy, sugar, high histamine foods, nightshades, salicylates, oxalates)?
- Are they more reactive after infections or flares?
- Do they eat differently when calm vs dysregulated?
- Are they avoiding food due to sensory issues, fear of pain, or OCD contamination fears?
- Are they eating compulsively? Our child had severe food OCD for a while.

You don't have to do it all at once. Start with what seems most obvious. Watch gently. Adjust slowly.

I highly recommend keeping a food log with notes to track reactions. It can be surprisingly helpful in identifying patterns that aren't immediately obvious.
I also highly recommend testing for immunological reactions to food through a **functional or integrative medicine practitioner**.
(Be aware that many conventional/allopathic doctors don't support this type of testing, and it's often not covered by insurance.)
And remember: this is not forever even if it feels like it.

Food grief and anxiety is real.

There may be days when your child sobs because they can't have a piece of birthday cake. When they stare at someone else's lunch and ask, "Why do I have to be the weird one?" When they feel excluded, punished, broken, just for having a body that reacts differently.

There may be days when you cry too because you wish you could just let them eat the damn cookie.

This is real grief. For them and for you. Let them grieve. Sit with them in it. And when you can, find joy in the little workarounds: a new recipe that doesn't hurt, a safe treat you make together, a picnic that feels almost normal. Even with restrictions, pleasure is still possible. And you are still doing a good job.

When They Won't Sleep

Nighttime Terror, Sleep Reversals, and the Hour You Start to Break

Sleep is where you're supposed to rest. But with PANS/PANDAS, nighttime becomes another battleground. They might be afraid to fall asleep, or afraid to be alone. They may beg you to stay, or rage when the lights go out. Sometimes they sleep all day and stay up all night, wired, haunted, unreachable. Other nights, they cry, twitch, shake, mutter nonsense.
And sometimes, they're just awake.
And so are you.
Night after night after night.

Anchoring Phrases (for Them)

- "Your body doesn't feel safe enough to sleep. That's not your fault."
- "I'll stay close until you feel calmer."
- "You are allowed to rest. There's no pressure to fall asleep right away."
- "Even if your brain is busy, your body can start to soften."
- "I believe your fear is real. And I'm not going anywhere."

Anchoring Phrases (for You, the Parent)

- "It's 4AM. No one is parenting well right now."
- "This is temporary. This will change. Someday this will just be a memory."
- "This isn't discipline failure. This is dysregulation."
- "It's okay to feel angry and exhausted and love them at the same time."

- "I am allowed to rest during the day. Rest is survival."
- "I am not responsible for fixing their sleep. I'm responsible for keeping them safe."

What Might Help (Some Nights)

- Weighted blankets, pillows, stuffed animals, or a calming scent
- Soft low music, brown noise/white noise, or rhythmic humming
- Movement before bed: a walk, stretching, or safe play
- A script you read aloud to cue safety: "Your bed is safe. This room is safe. Your body is healing. You are loved."
- Praying together, whether religious or not. We said a prayer to the angels from one of my child's favorite books.
- Letting go of the clock. Letting go of the fight. Focusing only on one calm breath at a time.
- Letting go of attachment to what the next day will bring.

Sleep may not come easy for them right now. But connection, safety, and nervous system quiet *can still happen*.

There is no one-size-fits-all solution for sleep with a PANS/PANDAS child. What works one week may stop working the next. What helps one family may backfire in yours. This is a process of compassionate trial and error.

Supportive Supplements & Medications
Always in consultation with a provider:

- GABA, L-theanine, or magnesium glycinate
- Antihistamines: Benadryl or hydroxyzine (especially for histamine-related flares)
- Herbs: Chinese skullcap and motherwort helped us, especially during agitated nights
- Benzodiazepines: Though not first-line, they can be life-saving in some flare states
- Psychiatric medications: SSRIs, antipsychotics, and sleep aids have helped some, but PANS kids often react paradoxically. Go slow. Watch carefully.

This is a nervous system in crisis, not a misbehaving child. And sometimes, the only way through the night is just making it through the night.

With all that said, if your child hasn't slept in a week and everyone in your house is ragged and fried, sometimes a trip to the ER can provide a much-needed reset.

In our case, it gave us access to medications we didn't have at home, and it helped interrupt the cycle just long enough for our child to get a little rest. I'm not recommending this across the board, and it's not without its own risks.

If you're considering it, tread carefully. Learn about your local hospitals and consult online parenting groups for personal experiences and insight. **Medical Gaslighting and Medical Kidnapping are very real.** Definitely educate yourself.

When Chemicals Don't Work the Way They're Supposed To

Why Some Things Help—and Others Hurt

One of the hardest lessons I've learned on this journey is that nothing is universal: not medications, not supplements, not even herbs that are supposedly "gentle."

Over the last five years, I tried everything. I amassed what felt like 500 bottles of capsules, powders, and tinctures. Each time someone said, "This helped my kid," I bought it. Each time a practitioner recommended something, I tried it. Sometimes it worked. Sometimes it backfired spectacularly.

A "helpful" anti-inflammatory supplement made things much worse. A calming remedy triggered rage. A trusted doctor prescribed something that sent us into chaos.

Eventually, I started looking deeper into how my kid's body actually processes chemicals. DNA SNPs, methylation pathways, neurotransmitter sensitivity, histamine load, detox capacity. I realized their system is not standard issue. Turmeric might be a miracle for one child and an absolute disaster for another.

How to Access Your Child's SNPs

You can get raw genetic data by using a direct-to-consumer DNA test like AncestryDNA or 23andMe. Once you've downloaded the raw file, upload it to a third-party analysis site. A functional medicine doctor or other doctor can also help you get this information.

Recommended: Sterling's App.This is a paid tool ($30–45) that offers a very detailed variant report, showing genes related to detox, methylation, neurotransmitters, immune system, and more. It's complex, but you can learn over time.

Other options include: Genetic Genie, SelfDecode and many others. This field keeps expanding.

These tools don't diagnose anything. They just show patterns. Interpretation takes time and often, trial and error.

Important: Some SNPs may explain why something that "helps most people" made your child worse. For example, turmeric increases dopamine. That's not good for everyone. Especially if your child is already overmethylated or prone to psychosis.

When Others Judge Your Parenting

You See a Child in Crisis. They See a Problem You Caused.

There is almost nothing as soul-crushing as showing up every day for a sick, suffering child and being judged for it.

You might hear:

"They just need discipline."

"Have you tried taking away screens?"

"If you didn't cater to them so much..."

"Back in my day, we didn't have all these labels."

You may be labeled a helicopter parent or told you're "too soft," "too enmeshed," or "coddling."

But the truth is:

You aren't trying to control them, you are trying to prevent catastrophe.

You know exactly how sensitive your child is. You know what will set them off in public. You have learned to read their body language like a barometer. And so you adapted. You make the choices you have to, often under pressure, often alone.

This is not a weakness. This is field medicine for a body under siege.

Most people judging you have no idea what they're talking about.

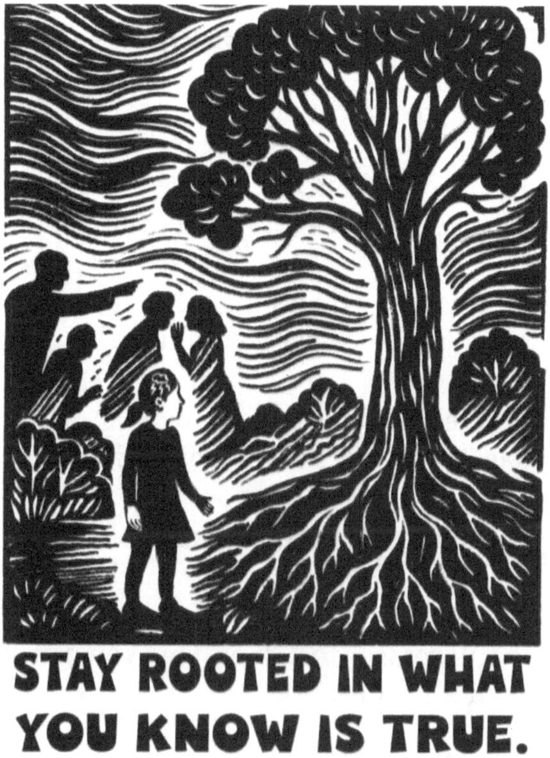

Anchoring Phrases (for Yourself)

- "They don't have to believe me for this to be real."
- "Their judgment is not more valid than my lived experience."
- "I have nothing to prove to people who haven't walked this path."
- "I don't owe calmness to people who meet me with cruelty."
- "I will keep choosing my child's safety over their approval."

If You're Still Trying to Explain

If you do feel up to educating someone:

"This is a neurological disorder caused by inflammation and immune dysfunction. It is not a behavior issue."

"We're following a treatment plan, but flares are unpredictable. Please be patient with us."

"Imagine your child changed overnight and no one believed you. That's what we're living with."

"It's okay if you don't understand. But please don't assume."

If someone still refuses to believe you, you can stop trying. Even if it's family.

Boundaries That Protect Your Sanity

- Stop updating people who only use the information against you.
- Say "we're going through a tough time" instead of justifying details.
- Don't invite commentary when you need privacy.
- Trust that your child doesn't need a perfect advocate, just a consistent one.
- You are not required to be palatable to people who are uncomfortable with suffering.
- You are allowed to protect your child, your energy, and your truth, even if no one else approves.

When Your Child Is in Rage or Psychosis

Explosive Behavior, Hallucinations, Delusions, or Wild Fear. This is the Brain on Fire.

This is when everything can feel unmanageable. Sometimes it IS unmanageable. It may look like screaming, violence, destruction, threats, or terrifying confusion. You might not recognize your child. The nervous system is completely hijacked by infection, inflammation, trauma, terror.
They are not in control. And neither are you.
But you can be the anchor, not by fixing it, but by regulating yourself and offering safety when they are untethered. This is very hard.

Anchoring Phrases (If You Can Speak Safely)

- Our mantra: "I am safe. I have time. I am loved." Choose your own version that resonates with your child.
- "I know this is scary. I'm not going to leave you.
- "I'm not your enemy. I'm your anchor. You can trust me."
- "This isn't who you are. This is something your brain is going through."
- "You are not in trouble. Your brain is inflamed. I know it's not your fault."
- "I'm going to stay calm for both of us right now."
- "We've survived this before. We can do it again."

Nonverbal Presence Ideas

- Sit on the ground to lower your height and reduce threat.
- Place your hand gently on your own chest or belly to demonstrate calm, not demand it.

- Keep your voice like a lullaby, even if they're yelling.
- Hum, rock, or offer a weighted object (if safe). Maybe your child will hum too. (Humming can stimulate the vagus nerve and activate the parasympathetic branch of the nervous system, which supports relaxation).
- If needed, exit the room to protect your own nervous system before returning with love.

Emergency Regulation Phrases for You (When You Feel Triggered or Afraid)

- "This is brain inflammation. Not personal."
- "My child is not the threat. Their flare is."
- "I can stay soft without collapsing."
- "I am allowed to walk away and still love them."
- "I will not match the storm. I will be the shore."

If your child is experiencing psychosis, you have no doubt considered an intervention like calling 911 or taking them to the ER. Sometimes you have no choice. We did it three times. Each time it was what I call a "pattern interrupt," but it did not solve the problem. If you are on the fence about this, I encourage you to join online parenting groups for PANS/ PANDAS and ask for advice. This is not an easy decision and it is especially hard when you're exhausted and fried, which I'm sure you are if you're dealing with this.

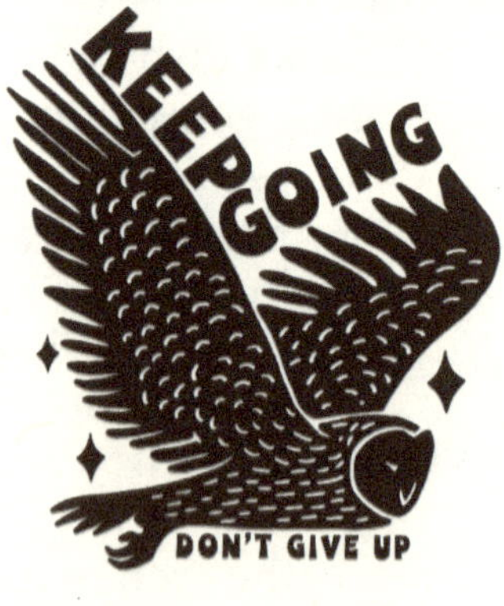

When Your Child Is Panicking or Flooded with Fear

Intrusive Thoughts, Terror, Catastrophic Thinking

This state often looks like terror, pacing, crying, obsessive questions, or begging for reassurance. You might hear things like: "Am I going to die?" "What if I lose control?" "What if I hurt you?" "What if I can't come back?" "What if I'm going to hell?"

These are not attention-seeking. They are fear-state loops caused by brain inflammation and nervous system chaos. It's not about reason. It's about survival. Your job is not to fix the thought. It's to help the body and brain feel safe enough to calm down.

Anchoring Phrases (Reassurance Without Over-Explaining)

- "Your brain is stuck in a scary loop. It's okay. We've seen this before."
- "That thought feels real, but it's not who you are."
- "You are safe. Even if it doesn't feel like it, you are safe."
- "You don't have to believe every thought your brain sends you."
- "It's okay to be scared. I'm right here. You're not alone."
- "You are not dangerous. You are overwhelmed."
- "You are a good person and worthy of love just like everyone."

Repetitive Question Traps

PANS/PANDAS kids often ask the same terrifying question over and over (e.g., "What if I never get better?") hoping for the exact right answer, but reassurance often feeds the loop. It can also become very frustrating. You may lose patience.

Instead of debating, try these responses:

- "That's a scary thought. Let's put it in the jar for now. You can come back to it later."
- "That's your flare talking. You don't have to solve it right now."
- "I believe you feel scared, but we don't need to answer that question today."
- "Let's breathe together instead of chasing that thought."

Calming the Nervous System

- Breathe in sync. Use your hand on your chest as a visual
- Offer cold water, peppermint tea, citrus essential oil to smell, or a soft or squishy object to hold.
- Use a mantra:
  "We are safe. This will pass."
  "This is not forever. It's just a temporary situation."
- Offer choice when possible: "Do you want to go outside or stay under the blanket?"
- If going outside is an option and there are trees, suggest hugging a tree. This is always grounding and calming for my kiddo. Alternatively, stand barefoot on the grass or dirt. This can also be grounding.
- If you're in the right space for it, you can gently place your hands on your child and offer them

calming, loving energy intentionally. Whether you call it Reiki, the Holy Spirit, Source, or simply love, that focused, heart-centered connection can be incredibly soothing. I'm not trying to be "woo woo" about it, just naming something that has helped us in hard moments. Sometimes, presence itself is medicine.

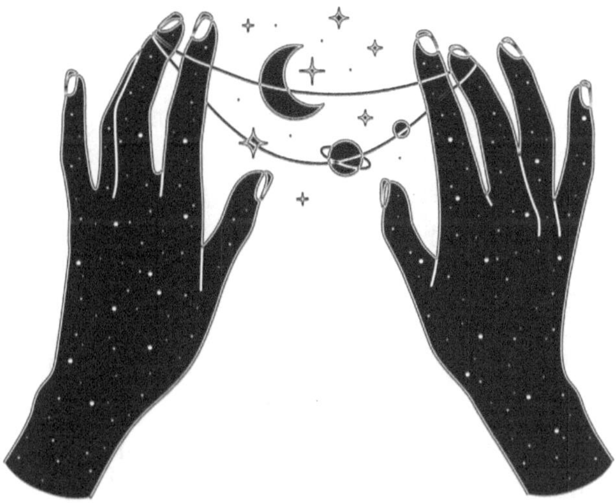

After the Storm: Repair and Recovery

When the Flare Calms, and You're Both Left Shaken

These moments can feel oddly quiet. Your child may come back to themselves, somewhat, or just seem exhausted. You might feel relief, or you might feel rage, grief, or numbness. This is often when your crash happens.

The truth is, post-crisis repair isn't about big conversations or life lessons. It's about reconnection, safety, thoughtful rituals, and giving both of you permission to feel whatever is there.

Anchoring Phrases for Reconnection

- "That was a really hard moment. I'm still here. We're okay."
- "Your brain went through something intense. You didn't do anything wrong."
- "We both got overwhelmed, but we're safe now."
- "It's okay if you don't remember everything. I love you the same."
- "You came back. That's what matters."
- "There's nothing you need to apologize for. Just rest."

Rituals of Repair (Small Acts That Say "We're Okay")

- Offer a favorite food or drink without fanfare.
- Sit together and watch something enjoyable, no talking required.
- Draw or color side-by-side.
- Say: "We made it through. Let's rest now."

- Light a candle, take a walk, or tidy up a small space together.
- Let yourself cry. Let them see your vulnerability, not your fear. Alternatively, it may frighten them if they see you cry. You know your child.
- Go for a drive to a place you both enjoy. For us, it was a spot called *Big Pocono,* the highest point in our area. We'd sit in the car, say nothing, and just look at the view. Over time, it became our reset button. You can find your own version of that place. It doesn't have to be far or fancy, just somewhere that feels quiet, safe, and a little bit outside the chaos.

For You, the Parent (Your Nervous System Matters Too)

- "That was too much. I am allowed to feel and acknowledge that."
- "I am going through something really hard. It's ok to just be."
- "I did what I could with the nervous system I had."
- "I can take 10 minutes now to come back to myself."
- "We are rebuilding safety together, one moment at a time."

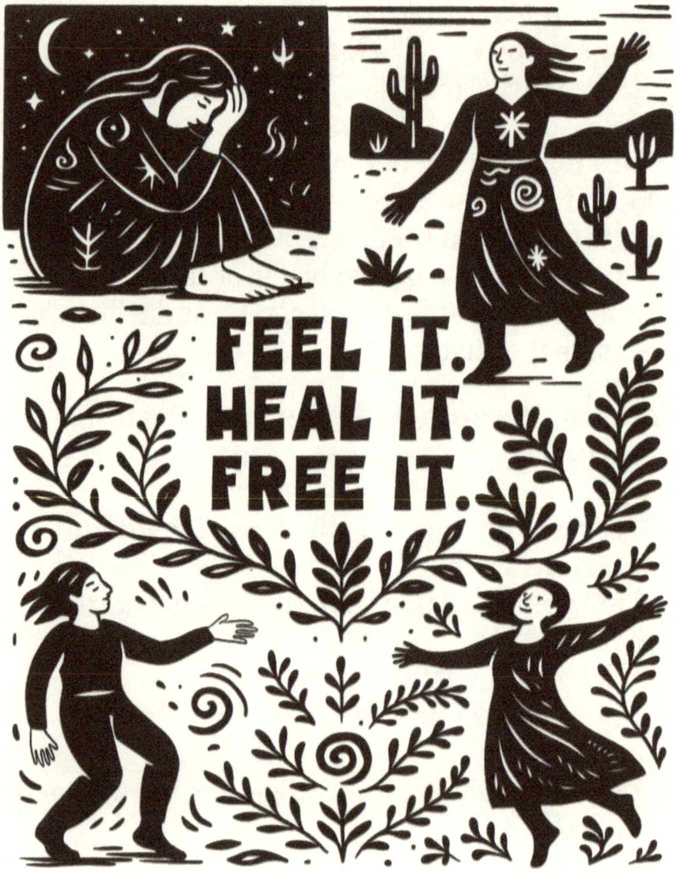
FEEL IT.
HEAL IT.
FREE IT.

When You Lose It: for the Parents Who've Snapped

For the Days You Yell, Slam Doors, Say Something You Regret, Break Down, or Worse

This illness can take you past the edge of what you thought you were capable of. You might do or say things you never imagined. You might scream. You might beg your child to stop. You might say "I can't do this anymore" or even "I don't want to live like this." You might break something, drive erratically. You might even do worse things.

If that's happened:
You are not a monster. You are not broken. You are in pain, and you are not alone.
The nervous system can only take so much. You are not failing, you are flaring, too.

Gentle Words for Yourself

- "That moment doesn't define me."
- "My nervous system hit its limit. That's not the same as being dangerous or unloving."
- "I can repair this. With myself, and with my child."
- "My child is sick, and I am surviving something extraordinary."
- "I don't have to be perfect. I just have to return to compassion."

If You Want to Repair (and You're Ready)

Children remember when their parents apologize. It creates trust.

- "I got overwhelmed. I yelled. I wish I hadn't. I still love you so much."
- "I'm not proud of how I acted. I'm working on it. You didn't cause it."
- "Even when I break down, I never stop loving you."
- "We're both going through something hard. We're going to keep trying."

You Deserve Support, Too

No one can do this alone, not well, not for long. If you snapped, it's not a sign of your weakness. It's a sign that your own system is overwhelmed, likely unsupported, possibly traumatized.

You don't need a personality overhaul. You need rest, compassion, maybe medication, probably therapy, definitely care.

You are a good parent doing a nearly impossible thing, and you're allowed to break down and still be a safe place for your child.

When You Need Something to Believe In

A Word About Faith, Spirit, and Survival

There will be days when your body is too exhausted to cry. When no one understands. When your child is screaming, or catatonic, or lost behind their eyes. On those days, you may ask:

What is holding me up?

If you have a faith lean on it.

Pray with all the raw honesty in your heart.

Yell at God. Whisper your pain to the angels. Light candles. Ask for grace. Ask for signs. Ask for help.

Let your faith hold what you cannot.

If you don't identify with any particular faith **find something that keeps your inner light from going out.**

- Sit under the sky and breathe.
- Move your body until it quiets your mind.
- Read something beautiful.
- Meditate. Scream into a pillow. Journal. Bury your face in the dog or cat.
- Let yoga or ritual or poetry or ancestors hold you.

And if that all feels too complex?

Binge a show, play Candy Crush, scroll mindlessly for a while, decorate a fake living room in Design Home, garden, run, play a sport, take up axe throwing. It might help to find online groups full of parents like you and post about your experience. There are some groups with parents who've been there and will support you with understanding and advice.

Also, sometimes, the only prayer you can manage is the one where you disassociate *just enough* to keep going. That counts.

Whatever helps you feel slightly lighter, slightly less alone, go toward that.
Find small moments of joy among the turmoil.
No shame. No rules. Breathe. Be Present. Let that be enough for now.

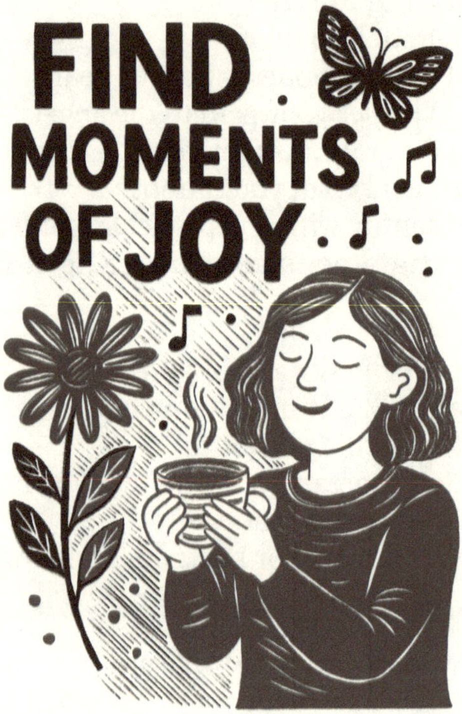

Mantras for the Ones Who Keep Going

For the Middle, the Aftermath, and the Days That Crack You Open

These are survival truths, anchors for parents who have faced hell and chosen to stay compassionate anyway. Take what you need. Leave the rest.

For the Middle of the Flare

- "I don't have control. But I have presence."
- "This is not who my child is. And this moment is not who I am either."
- "I am not required to fix this. I just need to hold the space and advocate."
- "His suffering is real. My sanity is important. I will address both as best I can."
- "The love I give her right now is enough, even if she can't feel it."
- "There is something holy about staying soft in the face of rage."

For the Hours After

- "That didn't feel survivable. And yet I survived it."
- "I am grieving someone who is still alive. That grief is real."
- "There's no perfect parent here. Just a wounded person doing their best."
- "I am not ashamed that I broke. I am proud that I came back."
- "He may not thank me. He may not understand. I am still choosing to love."
- "There is no finish line. But there are moments of peace. And I will find one."
- "I miss my freedom and my old life, but I have the strength to keep going and eventually find my way back to myself."

For Coming Back into Your Body (When You've Dissociated or Spiraled)

- Sit down. Touch the ground. Say: "This is the earth. It still holds me."
- Run water over your hands. Say: "This is real. This is now. That moment is over."
- Breathe and press your feet into the floor. Say: "I am in my body right now. I am not in the past or the future."
- Find one true thing in your environment: "The blanket is green. The air smells like dust. There's a bird outside."
- Lay your hand over your heart and say: "He/She is not alone. And neither am I."
- Cry over a glass of wine in the dark house after everyone else is asleep. (I have a vivid memory of doing this, and somehow it was cathartic, though it also felt terribly sad at the time).
- Find a time to drive alone, or just be alone and play loud music that you love.

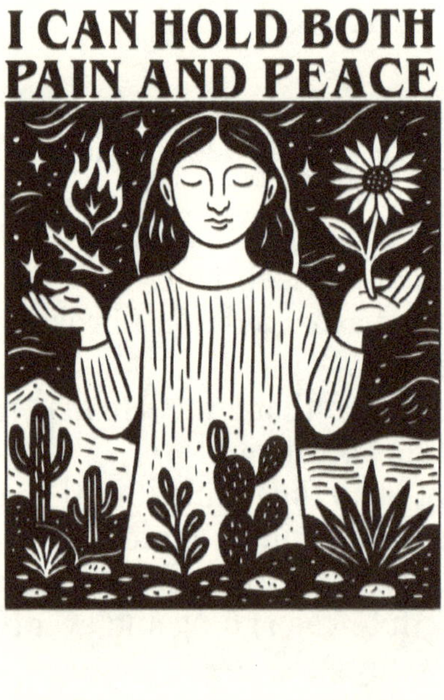

When Joy Disappears

PANS doesn't just take your child, it takes your whole household. It's not only the brain on fire, the OCD, the rage, the fear. It's the heaviness that settles over everyone. The laughter that stops. The spontaneity that vanishes. The relationships that wither under the pressure of pure survival.

For us, joy disappeared slowly at first, then suddenly it was gone. Misery and negativity seemed to take up permanent residence in my child's mind. It became the dominant energy in the house, and because I couldn't leave them, not physically, not emotionally, I was submerged in it too.

It was dark in more ways than one. Most nights, my kid was stuck in the bathroom, locked in OCD rituals that stretched for hours. I sat on the floor or paced the house, exhausted, scared, furious, helpless. We were up all night every night. We missed appointment after appointment because we had to sleep all day. The flipped circadian rhythm was inconvenient, even dangerous. It isolated us from the world and locked us in a reality that felt like it might never end. We lived in an inverted world where the only hours of peace came as the rest of the world was waking up.

For years, I lived in this state of upside-down isolation, exhausted, dysregulated, barely functioning. My world shrank to the dimensions of their illness. No holidays. No shared meals. No plans. No routine. No peace. I survived moment by moment. I couldn't think in days or weeks. I couldn't make plans. I lost friends.

But I could notice a single sip of espresso. I could let myself smile at my cat lying belly-up with her paws in the air. I could eat popcorn while binging a Netflix show at 3 a.m. I could feel a flicker of comfort and call that enough for the moment. These were survival practices.

Those moments didn't make it okay. We were not okay. But they reminded me that some part of me was still in there, still witnessing beauty, still reaching for the thread of light.

You don't have to find peace. You don't have to feel grateful. But if anything small breaks through, something silly, warm, sweet, or soft, recognize it. Let it remind you that you're still present and alive in this too.

We lived in Pennsylvania during the hardest years, and dawn there is magical. It became a strange, sacred time for me. Painful and beautiful. A threshold I crossed every day, weary but still standing. Every day being awake until dawn reminded me how far off we were from normal life, but it also held beauty I couldn't ignore: mist curling over the hills, cool air whispering through the trees, deer moving silently through the yard like spirits. It was haunting and beautiful. A thread of softness in a life that had become unbearably hard.

I learned not to wait for big joy. Just a moment. A spark. A breath. The warmth of a blanket. A funny meme. A sunrise. Joy wasn't a destination, it was a thread. Sometimes thin, sometimes strong. But always there, if I was willing to notice.

This illness has a way of making everything feel impossible: joy, ease, connection, lightness. I want to mention that, because people don't talk about it enough. We talk about symptoms. We talk about flares. But we don't always say: **this can hollow out your life.**

If you feel like joy has been stolen from your home, you are not alone. You are not doing it wrong. That is what this illness can do, but it can also shift even if it's been years, even if you think it never will.

Don't give up looking for moments of beauty, for a flicker of light, for something that reminds you that you're still in there too.

At a routine checkup in my late 40s, my doctor gave me a depression screening. I'd never taken anything before, no meds, no diagnosis, but I was clinically depressed. I started an antidepressant, and it helped. It didn't fix the situation, but it gave me enough motivation to keep going.

Needing help, medical help, psychiatric help, chemical help, is not a failure. It doesn't mean you're weak or broken. It means your body and mind are trying to survive an impossible situation.

We don't talk enough about caregiver depression, about how deeply it cuts when you're chronically witnessing suffering and danger and losing your sense of self. But it's real. It happened to me. And I'm still here.

Let this be your permission slip: to grieve, to ask for help, to medicate if needed, to name the joy that's been stolen, and to still look for pieces of it wherever you can.

It might help to intentionally reflect on things that brought you joy in the past week. This isn't a gratitude journal. This is just a grounding exercise to help you survive. What small thing brought you a flicker of comfort this week? It doesn't have to be profound.

It can be your beloved pet.

It can be food. It can be a breeze.

It can be a dumb joke, or the way light came through the window.

Let that thread remind you: you are still here.

"There is a crack in everything. That's how the light gets in."
– Leonard Cohen

Sometimes the thread is barely visible.

But it's there, a sliver of light breaking through the cracks.

Let yourself notice it, even if you're exhausted, even if you're angry, even if things feel hopeless. The light still knows how to find you.

Final Thoughts

If you're reading this, it's because you care deeply and you're doing your best, often under extreme pressure and isolation. This path can feel overwhelming, but you are not alone. There are thousands of families walking this road too, fighting to be heard, trying every angle, and holding their children through the storm.

Whether your days are filled with research and therapies, or just surviving one moment to the next, please remember: your love is essential, your intuition matters, your efforts, even the unseen, exhausted ones count.

Keep reaching for the light, keep trusting that healing is possible, even when it's slow or nonlinear. And when you need to fall apart, that's okay too. There is no perfect way to parent through this. There is only love, persistence, and the slow unfolding of your child's journey back to themselves.

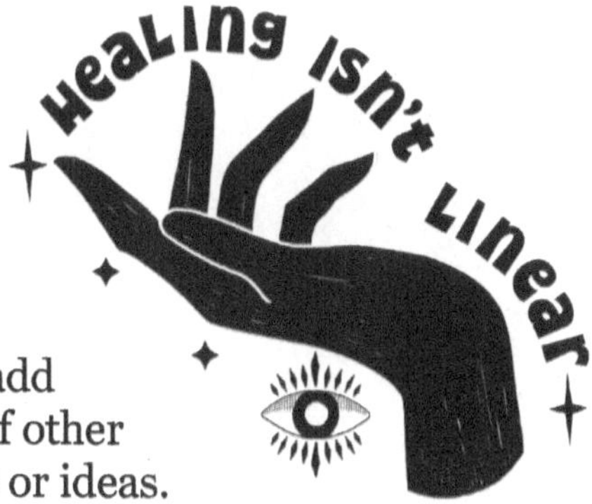

There's so much more I could say. This little book only scratches the surface of everything I've learned and everything we've lived through this illness. I may add more over time, especially if other parents share their insights or ideas.

If you'd like to be notified when I make updates, or when I release more resources, like worksheets, journal pages, or future books, head over to: junipermoon.kit.com/mailinglist and **join my mailing list**. You can also email me at info@junipermooncolors.com

Please also visit my Etsy store where I will be adding useful printables like symptom trackers if that is useful for you!

https://www.etsy.com/shop/JuniperMoonColors

Resources and Support

Here are some trusted websites to deepen your understanding and find community:

PANDAS Network
https://pandasnetwork.org
Offers research, treatment information, stories, and resources for families.

PANDAS Physicians Network (PPN)
https://www.pandasppn.org
A resource for finding PANS/PANDAS-aware doctors and clinical guidelines.

Neuroimmune Foundation
https://neuroimmune.org
Focuses on education, outreach, and research around neuroimmune disorders including PANS/PANDAS.

The Autoimmune Association
https://autoimmune.org/
The Autoimmune Association is the world's leading nonprofit organization dedicated to autoimmune awareness, advocacy, education, and research.

ASPIRE (Alliance to Solve PANS & Immune-Related Encephalopathies)
https://aspire.care
Includes educational materials, advocacy tools, and webinars for caregivers and providers.

The PARENTS of CHILDREN with PANDAS/ PANS/LYME/TICK-BORNE DISEASES Facebook Group

A large peer-support group for sharing stories, questions, and tips.

The PANDAS PARENTS Facebook Group

A large peer-support group for sharing stories, questions, and tips.

(Both groups are searchable on Facebook)

There are many Facebook groups. I recommend joining whichever ones resonate for you.

www.ingramcontent.com/pod-product-compliance
Lightning Source LLC
LaVergne TN
LVHW090432210926
848480LV00002B/799
9798233769221